Anxiety Journal

INFORMATIONS

NAME

ADDRESS

E-MAIL ADDRESS

WEBSITE

PHONE   **FAX**

EMERGENCY CONTACT PERSON

PHONE   **FAX**

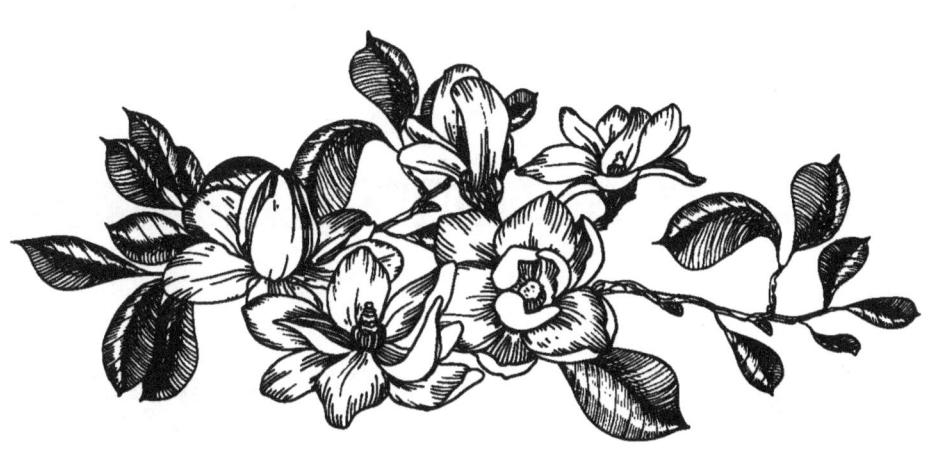

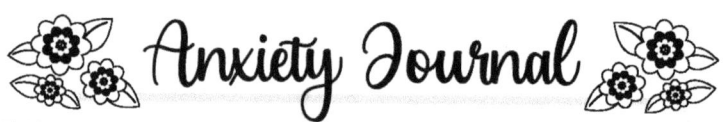

Anxiety Journal

DATE .... TIME ....

PLACE .... SOURCE OF ANXIETY ....

PHYSICAL SENSATIONS ....

NEGATIVE BELIEVES

ABOUT SITUATION ....
....

ABOUT YOUSELF ....
....

WHAT FACTS DO YOU KNOW ARE TRUE?

ABOUT SITUATION ....
....

ABOUT YOUSELF ....
....

WHAT HAPPENED?

....
....

HOW DID IT MAKE YOU FEEL?

....
....

HOW DID YOU REACT?

....
....

WHAT HELPS YOU SOOTHE YOUR ANXIETY?

....
....

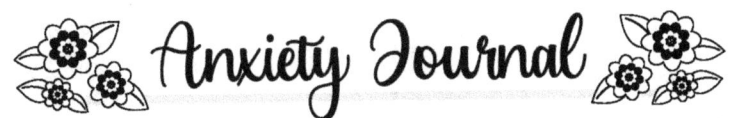

Anxiety Journal

DATE .... **TIME** ....

PLACE .... **SOURCE OF ANXIETY** ....

PHYSICAL SENSATIONS ....

NEGATIVE BELIEVES

ABOUT SITUATION ....

....

ABOUT YOUSELF ....

....

WHAT FACTS DO YOU KNOW ARE TRUE?

ABOUT SITUATION ....

....

ABOUT YOUSELF ....

....

WHAT HAPPENED?

....

....

HOW DID IT MAKE YOU FEEL?

....

....

HOW DID YOU REACT?

....

....

WHAT HELPS YOU SOOTHE YOUR ANXIETY?

....

....

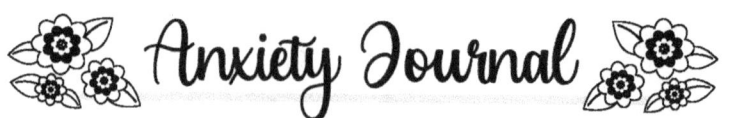

Anxiety Journal

DATE .... TIME ....

PLACE .... SOURCE OF ANXIETY ....

PHYSICAL SENSATIONS ....

NEGATIVE BELIEVES

ABOUT SITUATION ....
....

ABOUT YOUSELF ....
....

WHAT FACTS DO YOU KNOW ARE TRUE?

ABOUT SITUATION ....
....

ABOUT YOUSELF ....
....

WHAT HAPPENED?

....
....

HOW DID IT MAKE YOU FEEL?

....
....

HOW DID YOU REACT?

....
....

WHAT HELPS YOU SOOTHE YOUR ANXIETY?

....
....

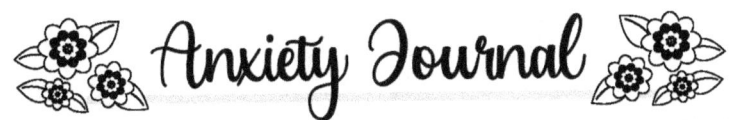

Anxiety Journal

DATE .... **TIME** ....

PLACE .... **SOURCE OF ANXIETY** ....

PHYSICAL SENSATIONS ....

NEGATIVE BELIEVES

ABOUT SITUATION ....

....

ABOUT YOUSELF ....

....

WHAT FACTS DO YOU KNOW ARE TRUE?

ABOUT SITUATION ....

....

ABOUT YOUSELF ....

....

WHAT HAPPENED?

....

....

HOW DID IT MAKE YOU FEEL?

....

....

HOW DID YOU REACT?

....

....

WHAT HELPS YOU SOOTHE YOUR ANXIETY?

....

....

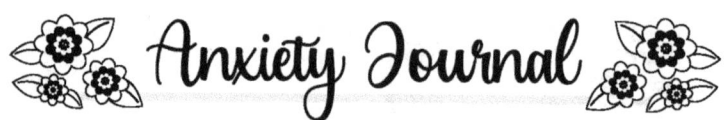

Anxiety Journal

DATE .... TIME ....

PLACE .... SOURCE OF ANXIETY ....

PHYSICAL SENSATIONS ....

NEGATIVE BELIEVES

ABOUT SITUATION ....

....

ABOUT YOUSELF ....

....

WHAT FACTS DO YOU KNOW ARE TRUE?

ABOUT SITUATION ....

....

ABOUT YOUSELF ....

....

WHAT HAPPENED?

....

....

HOW DID IT MAKE YOU FEEL?

....

....

HOW DID YOU REACT?

....

....

WHAT HELPS YOU SOOTHE YOUR ANXIETY?

....

....

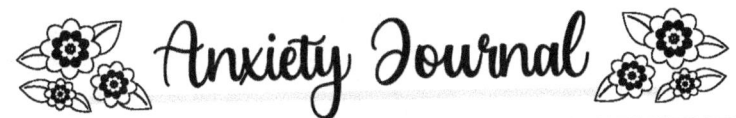

Anxiety Journal

DATE .... **TIME** ....

PLACE .... **SOURCE OF ANXIETY** ....

PHYSICAL SENSATIONS ....

NEGATIVE BELIEVES

ABOUT SITUATION ....
....

ABOUT YOUSELF ....
....

WHAT FACTS DO YOU KNOW ARE TRUE?

ABOUT SITUATION ....
....

ABOUT YOUSELF ....
....

WHAT HAPPENED?

....
....

HOW DID IT MAKE YOU FEEL?

....
....

HOW DID YOU REACT?

....
....

WHAT HELPS YOU SOOTHE YOUR ANXIETY?

....
....

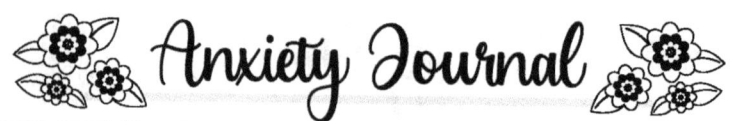

Anxiety Journal

DATE .... TIME ....

PLACE .... SOURCE OF ANXIETY ....

PHYSICAL SENSATIONS ....

NEGATIVE BELIEVES

ABOUT SITUATION ....

....

ABOUT YOUSELF ....

....

WHAT FACTS DO YOU KNOW ARE TRUE?

ABOUT SITUATION ....

....

ABOUT YOUSELF ....

....

WHAT HAPPENED?

....

....

HOW DID IT MAKE YOU FEEL?

....

....

HOW DID YOU REACT?

....

....

WHAT HELPS YOU SOOTHE YOUR ANXIETY?

....

....

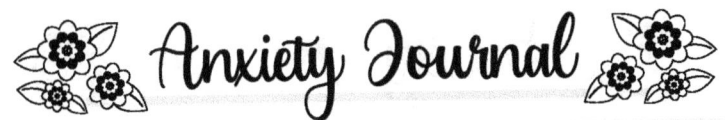

Anxiety Journal

DATE _____ TIME _____

PLACE _____ SOURCE OF ANXIETY _____

PHYSICAL SENSATIONS _____

NEGATIVE BELIEVES

ABOUT SITUATION ....

....

ABOUT YOUSELF ....

....

WHAT FACTS DO YOU KNOW ARE TRUE?

ABOUT SITUATION ....

....

ABOUT YOUSELF ....

....

WHAT HAPPENED?

....

....

HOW DID IT MAKE YOU FEEL?

....

....

HOW DID YOU REACT?

....

....

WHAT HELPS YOU SOOTHE YOUR ANXIETY?

....

....

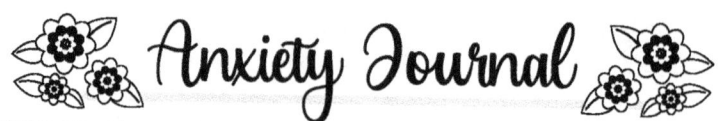

Anxiety Journal

DATE .... **TIME** ....

PLACE .... **SOURCE OF ANXIETY** ....

PHYSICAL SENSATIONS ....

NEGATIVE BELIEVES

ABOUT SITUATION ....
....

ABOUT YOUSELF ....
....

WHAT FACTS DO YOU KNOW ARE TRUE?

ABOUT SITUATION ....
....

ABOUT YOUSELF ....
....

WHAT HAPPENED?

....
....

HOW DID IT MAKE YOU FEEL?

....
....

HOW DID YOU REACT?

....
....

WHAT HELPS YOU SOOTHE YOUR ANXIETY?

....
....

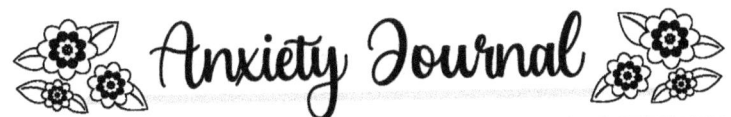

Anxiety Journal

DATE .... TIME ....

PLACE .... SOURCE OF ANXIETY ....

PHYSICAL SENSATIONS ....

NEGATIVE BELIEVES

ABOUT SITUATION ....

....

ABOUT YOUSELF ....

....

WHAT FACTS DO YOU KNOW ARE TRUE?

ABOUT SITUATION ....

....

ABOUT YOUSELF ....

....

WHAT HAPPENED?

....

....

HOW DID IT MAKE YOU FEEL?

....

....

HOW DID YOU REACT?

....

....

WHAT HELPS YOU SOOTHE YOUR ANXIETY?

....

....

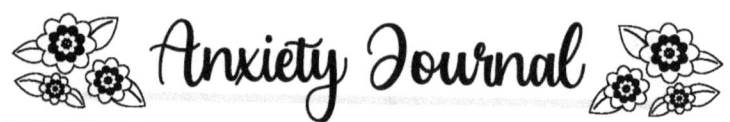

Anxiety Journal

DATE .... **TIME** ....

PLACE .... **SOURCE OF ANXIETY** ....

PHYSICAL SENSATIONS ....

NEGATIVE BELIEVES

ABOUT SITUATION ....
....

ABOUT YOUSELF ....
....

WHAT FACTS DO YOU KNOW ARE TRUE?

ABOUT SITUATION ....
....

ABOUT YOUSELF ....
....

WHAT HAPPENED?

....
....

HOW DID IT MAKE YOU FEEL?

....
....

HOW DID YOU REACT?

....
....

WHAT HELPS YOU SOOTHE YOUR ANXIETY?

....
....

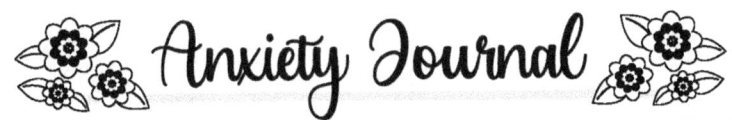

Anxiety Journal

DATE _____ **TIME** _____

PLACE _____ **SOURCE OF ANXIETY** _____

PHYSICAL SENSATIONS _____

NEGATIVE BELIEVES

ABOUT SITUATION ....

....

ABOUT YOUSELF ....

....

WHAT FACTS DO YOU KNOW ARE TRUE?

ABOUT SITUATION ....

....

ABOUT YOUSELF ....

....

WHAT HAPPENED?

....

....

HOW DID IT MAKE YOU FEEL?

....

....

HOW DID YOU REACT?

....

....

WHAT HELPS YOU SOOTHE YOUR ANXIETY?

....

....

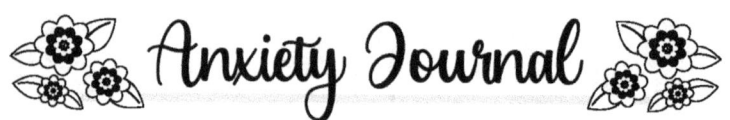
Anxiety Journal

DATE   **TIME**

PLACE   **SOURCE OF ANXIETY**

PHYSICAL SENSATIONS

NEGATIVE BELIEVES

ABOUT SITUATION ....
....

ABOUT YOUSELF ....
....

WHAT FACTS DO YOU KNOW ARE TRUE?

ABOUT SITUATION ....
....

ABOUT YOUSELF ....
....

WHAT HAPPENED?

....
....

HOW DID IT MAKE YOU FEEL?

....
....

HOW DID YOU REACT?

....
....

WHAT HELPS YOU SOOTHE YOUR ANXIETY?

....
....

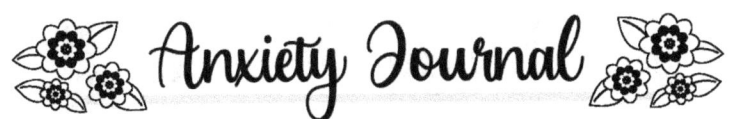

Anxiety Journal

DATE   **TIME**

PLACE   **SOURCE OF ANXIETY**

PHYSICAL SENSATIONS

NEGATIVE BELIEVES

ABOUT SITUATION ....

....

ABOUT YOUSELF ....

....

WHAT FACTS DO YOU KNOW ARE TRUE?

ABOUT SITUATION ....

....

ABOUT YOUSELF ....

....

WHAT HAPPENED?

....

....

HOW DID IT MAKE YOU FEEL?

....

....

HOW DID YOU REACT?

....

....

WHAT HELPS YOU SOOTHE YOUR ANXIETY?

....

....

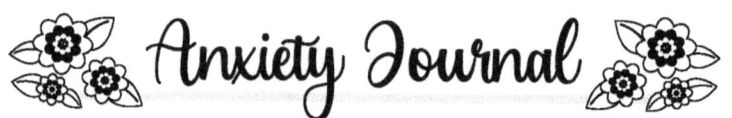

Anxiety Journal

DATE .... **TIME**

PLACE .... **SOURCE OF ANXIETY**

PHYSICAL SENSATIONS ....

NEGATIVE BELIEVES

ABOUT SITUATION ....
....

ABOUT YOUSELF ....
....

WHAT FACTS DO YOU KNOW ARE TRUE?

ABOUT SITUATION ....
....

ABOUT YOUSELF ....
....

WHAT HAPPENED?

....
....

HOW DID IT MAKE YOU FEEL?

....
....

HOW DID YOU REACT?

....
....

WHAT HELPS YOU SOOTHE YOUR ANXIETY?

....
....

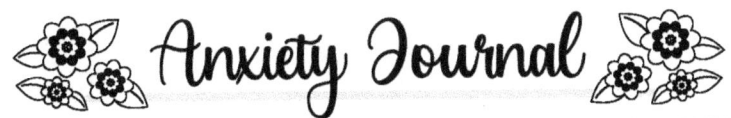

Anxiety Journal

DATE .... **TIME** ....

PLACE .... **SOURCE OF ANXIETY** ....

PHYSICAL SENSATIONS ....

NEGATIVE BELIEVES

ABOUT SITUATION ....

....

ABOUT YOUSELF ....

....

WHAT FACTS DO YOU KNOW ARE TRUE?

ABOUT SITUATION ....

....

ABOUT YOUSELF ....

....

WHAT HAPPENED?

....

....

HOW DID IT MAKE YOU FEEL?

....

....

HOW DID YOU REACT?

....

....

WHAT HELPS YOU SOOTHE YOUR ANXIETY?

....

....

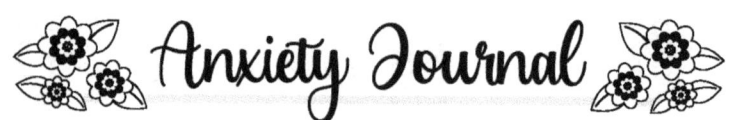

Anxiety Journal

DATE .... **TIME** ....

PLACE .... **SOURCE OF ANXIETY** ....

PHYSICAL SENSATIONS ....

NEGATIVE BELIEVES

ABOUT SITUATION ....
....

ABOUT YOUSELF ....
....

WHAT FACTS DO YOU KNOW ARE TRUE?

ABOUT SITUATION ....
....

ABOUT YOUSELF ....
....

WHAT HAPPENED?

....
....

HOW DID IT MAKE YOU FEEL?

....
....

HOW DID YOU REACT?

....
....

WHAT HELPS YOU SOOTHE YOUR ANXIETY?

....
....

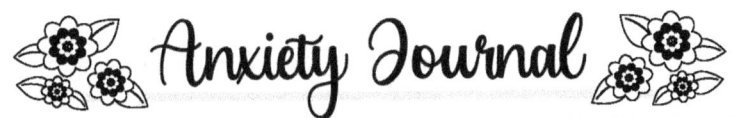

Anxiety Journal

DATE _____   **TIME** _____

PLACE _____   **SOURCE OF ANXIETY** _____

PHYSICAL SENSATIONS _____

NEGATIVE BELIEVES

ABOUT SITUATION ....

....

ABOUT YOUSELF ....

....

WHAT FACTS DO YOU KNOW ARE TRUE?

ABOUT SITUATION ....

....

ABOUT YOUSELF ....

....

WHAT HAPPENED?

....

....

HOW DID IT MAKE YOU FEEL?

....

....

HOW DID YOU REACT?

....

....

WHAT HELPS YOU SOOTHE YOUR ANXIETY?

....

....

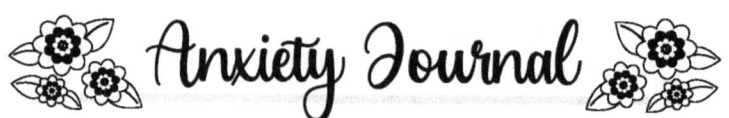
Anxiety Journal

DATE .... **TIME** ....

PLACE .... **SOURCE OF ANXIETY** ....

PHYSICAL SENSATIONS ....

NEGATIVE BELIEVES

ABOUT SITUATION ....

....

ABOUT YOUSELF ....

....

WHAT FACTS DO YOU KNOW ARE TRUE?

ABOUT SITUATION ....

....

ABOUT YOUSELF ....

....

WHAT HAPPENED?

....

....

HOW DID IT MAKE YOU FEEL?

....

....

HOW DID YOU REACT?

....

....

WHAT HELPS YOU SOOTHE YOUR ANXIETY?

....

....

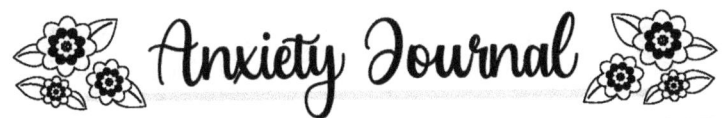# Anxiety Journal

DATE   **TIME**

PLACE   **SOURCE OF ANXIETY**

PHYSICAL SENSATIONS

NEGATIVE BELIEVES

ABOUT SITUATION ....

....

ABOUT YOUSELF ....

....

WHAT FACTS DO YOU KNOW ARE TRUE?

ABOUT SITUATION ....

....

ABOUT YOUSELF ....

....

WHAT HAPPENED?

....

....

HOW DID IT MAKE YOU FEEL?

....

....

HOW DID YOU REACT?

....

....

WHAT HELPS YOU SOOTHE YOUR ANXIETY?

....

....

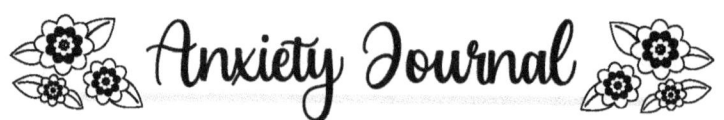

Anxiety Journal

DATE _____   **TIME** _____

PLACE _____   **SOURCE OF ANXIETY** _____

PHYSICAL SENSATIONS _____

NEGATIVE BELIEVES

ABOUT SITUATION ....
....

ABOUT YOURSELF ....
....

WHAT FACTS DO YOU KNOW ARE TRUE?

ABOUT SITUATION ....
....

ABOUT YOUSELF ....
....

WHAT HAPPENED?

....
....

HOW DID IT MAKE YOU FEEL?

....
....

HOW DID YOU REACT?

....
....

WHAT HELPS YOU SOOTHE YOUR ANXIETY?

....
....

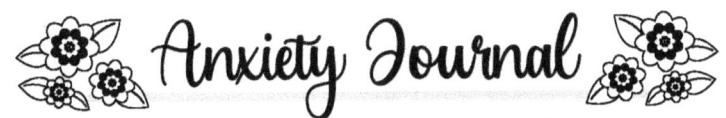
Anxiety Journal

DATE _____   **TIME** _____

PLACE _____   **SOURCE OF ANXIETY** _____

PHYSICAL SENSATIONS _____

NEGATIVE BELIEVES

ABOUT SITUATION ....

....

ABOUT YOUSELF ....

....

WHAT FACTS DO YOU KNOW ARE TRUE?

ABOUT SITUATION ....

....

ABOUT YOUSELF ....

....

WHAT HAPPENED?

....

....

HOW DID IT MAKE YOU FEEL?

....

....

HOW DID YOU REACT?

....

....

WHAT HELPS YOU SOOTHE YOUR ANXIETY?

....

....

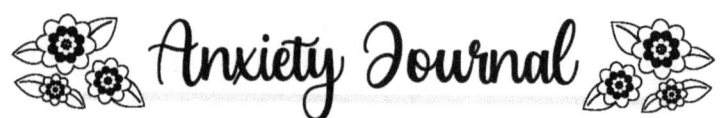

Anxiety Journal

DATE .... **TIME**

PLACE .... **SOURCE OF ANXIETY**

PHYSICAL SENSATIONS ....

NEGATIVE BELIEVES

ABOUT SITUATION ....
....

ABOUT YOUSELF ....
....

WHAT FACTS DO YOU KNOW ARE TRUE?

ABOUT SITUATION ....
....

ABOUT YOUSELF ....
....

WHAT HAPPENED?

....
....

HOW DID IT MAKE YOU FEEL?

....
....

HOW DID YOU REACT?

....
....

WHAT HELPS YOU SOOTHE YOUR ANXIETY?

....
....

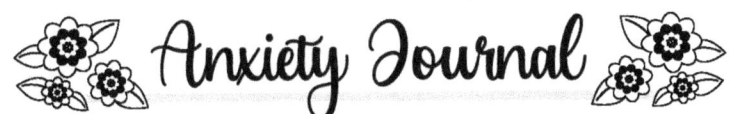

Anxiety Journal

DATE

TIME

PLACE

SOURCE OF ANXIETY

PHYSICAL SENSATIONS

NEGATIVE BELIEVES

ABOUT SITUATION ....

....

ABOUT YOUSELF ....

....

WHAT FACTS DO YOU KNOW ARE TRUE?

ABOUT SITUATION ....

....

ABOUT YOUSELF ....

....

WHAT HAPPENED?

....

....

HOW DID IT MAKE YOU FEEL?

....

....

HOW DID YOU REACT?

....

....

WHAT HELPS YOU SOOTHE YOUR ANXIETY?

....

....

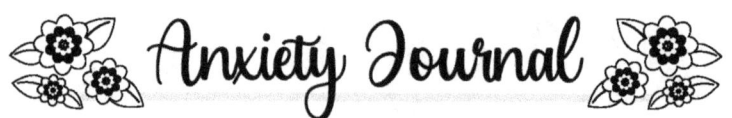

Anxiety Journal

DATE   **TIME**

PLACE   **SOURCE OF ANXIETY**

PHYSICAL SENSATIONS

NEGATIVE BELIEVES

ABOUT SITUATION ....
....

ABOUT YOUSELF ....
....

WHAT FACTS DO YOU KNOW ARE TRUE?

ABOUT SITUATION ....
....

ABOUT YOUSELF ....
....

WHAT HAPPENED?

....
....

HOW DID IT MAKE YOU FEEL?

....
....

HOW DID YOU REACT?

....
....

WHAT HELPS YOU SOOTHE YOUR ANXIETY?

....
....

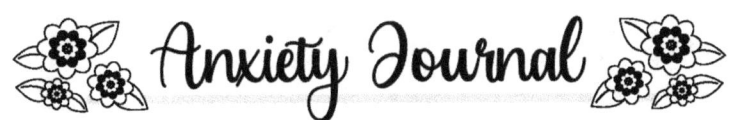

Anxiety Journal

DATE .... **TIME** ....

PLACE .... **SOURCE OF ANXIETY** ....

PHYSICAL SENSATIONS ....

NEGATIVE BELIEVES

ABOUT SITUATION ....

....

ABOUT YOUSELF ....

....

WHAT FACTS DO YOU KNOW ARE TRUE?

ABOUT SITUATION ....

....

ABOUT YOUSELF ....

....

WHAT HAPPENED?

....

....

HOW DID IT MAKE YOU FEEL?

....

....

HOW DID YOU REACT?

....

....

WHAT HELPS YOU SOOTHE YOUR ANXIETY?

....

....

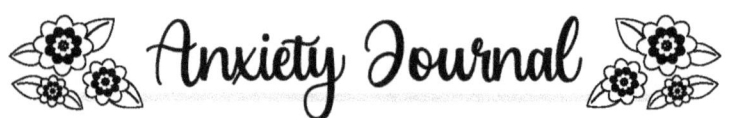# Anxiety Journal

DATE

TIME

PLACE

SOURCE OF ANXIETY

PHYSICAL SENSATIONS

NEGATIVE BELIEVES

ABOUT SITUATION ....

....

ABOUT YOUSELF ....

....

WHAT FACTS DO YOU KNOW ARE TRUE?

ABOUT SITUATION ....

....

ABOUT YOUSELF ....

....

WHAT HAPPENED?

....

....

HOW DID IT MAKE YOU FEEL?

....

....

HOW DID YOU REACT?

....

....

WHAT HELPS YOU SOOTHE YOUR ANXIETY?

....

....

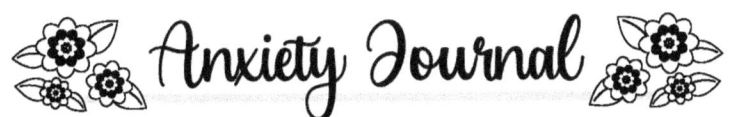
Anxiety Journal

DATE .... **TIME** ....

PLACE .... **SOURCE OF ANXIETY** ....

PHYSICAL SENSATIONS ....

NEGATIVE BELIEVES

ABOUT SITUATION ....

....

ABOUT YOUSELF ....

....

WHAT FACTS DO YOU KNOW ARE TRUE?

ABOUT SITUATION ....

....

ABOUT YOUSELF ....

....

WHAT HAPPENED?

....

....

HOW DID IT MAKE YOU FEEL?

....

....

HOW DID YOU REACT?

....

....

WHAT HELPS YOU SOOTHE YOUR ANXIETY?

....

....

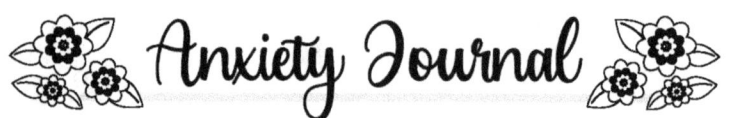

Anxiety Journal

DATE .... **TIME** ....

PLACE .... **SOURCE OF ANXIETY** ....

PHYSICAL SENSATIONS ....

NEGATIVE BELIEVES

ABOUT SITUATION ....

....

ABOUT YOUSELF ....

....

WHAT FACTS DO YOU KNOW ARE TRUE?

ABOUT SITUATION ....

....

ABOUT YOUSELF ....

....

WHAT HAPPENED?

....

....

HOW DID IT MAKE YOU FEEL?

....

....

HOW DID YOU REACT?

....

....

WHAT HELPS YOU SOOTHE YOUR ANXIETY?

....

....

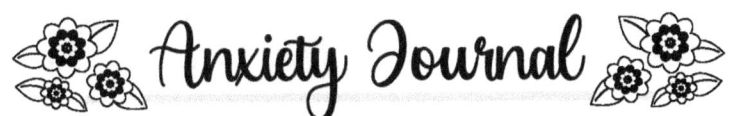

Anxiety Journal

DATE .... **TIME** ....

PLACE .... **SOURCE OF ANXIETY** ....

PHYSICAL SENSATIONS ....

NEGATIVE BELIEVES

ABOUT SITUATION ....
....

ABOUT YOUSELF ....
....

WHAT FACTS DO YOU KNOW ARE TRUE?

ABOUT SITUATION ....
....

ABOUT YOUSELF ....
....

WHAT HAPPENED?

....
....

HOW DID IT MAKE YOU FEEL?

....
....

HOW DID YOU REACT?

....
....

WHAT HELPS YOU SOOTHE YOUR ANXIETY?

....
....

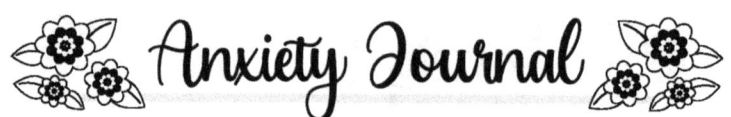

Anxiety Journal

DATE .... **TIME** ....

PLACE .... **SOURCE OF ANXIETY** ....

PHYSICAL SENSATIONS ....

NEGATIVE BELIEVES

ABOUT SITUATION ....
....

ABOUT YOUSELF ....
....

WHAT FACTS DO YOU KNOW ARE TRUE?

ABOUT SITUATION ....
....

ABOUT YOUSELF ....
....

WHAT HAPPENED?

....
....

HOW DID IT MAKE YOU FEEL?

....
....

HOW DID YOU REACT?

....
....

WHAT HELPS YOU SOOTHE YOUR ANXIETY?

....
....

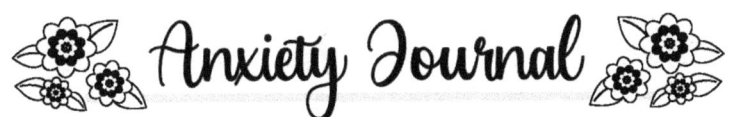

Anxiety Journal

DATE .... **TIME** ....

PLACE .... **SOURCE OF ANXIETY** ....

PHYSICAL SENSATIONS ....

NEGATIVE BELIEVES

ABOUT SITUATION ....
....

ABOUT YOUSELF ....
....

WHAT FACTS DO YOU KNOW ARE TRUE?

ABOUT SITUATION ....
....

ABOUT YOUSELF ....
....

WHAT HAPPENED?

....
....

HOW DID IT MAKE YOU FEEL?

....
....

HOW DID YOU REACT?

....
....

WHAT HELPS YOU SOOTHE YOUR ANXIETY?

....
....

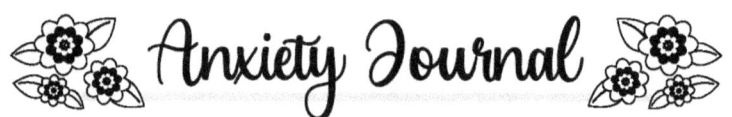

Anxiety Journal

DATE .... **TIME** ....

PLACE .... **SOURCE OF ANXIETY** ....

PHYSICAL SENSATIONS ....

NEGATIVE BELIEVES

ABOUT SITUATION ....
....

ABOUT YOUSELF ....
....

WHAT FACTS DO YOU KNOW ARE TRUE?

ABOUT SITUATION ....
....

ABOUT YOUSELF ....
....

WHAT HAPPENED?

....
....

HOW DID IT MAKE YOU FEEL?

....
....

HOW DID YOU REACT?

....
....

WHAT HELPS YOU SOOTHE YOUR ANXIETY?

....
....

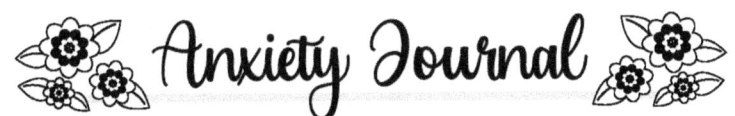

Anxiety Journal

DATE .... **TIME** ....

PLACE .... **SOURCE OF ANXIETY** ....

PHYSICAL SENSATIONS ....

NEGATIVE BELIEVES

ABOUT SITUATION ....

....

ABOUT YOUSELF ....

....

WHAT FACTS DO YOU KNOW ARE TRUE?

ABOUT SITUATION ....

....

ABOUT YOUSELF ....

....

WHAT HAPPENED?

....

....

HOW DID IT MAKE YOU FEEL?

....

....

HOW DID YOU REACT?

....

....

WHAT HELPS YOU SOOTHE YOUR ANXIETY?

....

....

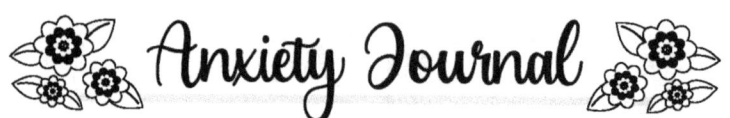

Anxiety Journal

DATE .... TIME ....

PLACE .... SOURCE OF ANXIETY ....

PHYSICAL SENSATIONS ....

NEGATIVE BELIEVES

ABOUT SITUATION ....

....

ABOUT YOUSELF ....

....

WHAT FACTS DO YOU KNOW ARE TRUE?

ABOUT SITUATION ....

....

ABOUT YOUSELF ....

....

WHAT HAPPENED?

....

....

HOW DID IT MAKE YOU FEEL?

....

....

HOW DID YOU REACT?

....

....

WHAT HELPS YOU SOOTHE YOUR ANXIETY?

....

....

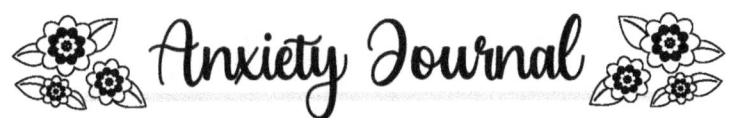

Anxiety Journal

DATE   **TIME**

PLACE   **SOURCE OF ANXIETY**

PHYSICAL SENSATIONS

NEGATIVE BELIEVES

ABOUT SITUATION ....

....

ABOUT YOUSELF ....

....

WHAT FACTS DO YOU KNOW ARE TRUE?

ABOUT SITUATION ....

....

ABOUT YOUSELF ....

....

WHAT HAPPENED?

....

....

HOW DID IT MAKE YOU FEEL?

....

....

HOW DID YOU REACT?

....

....

WHAT HELPS YOU SOOTHE YOUR ANXIETY?

....

....

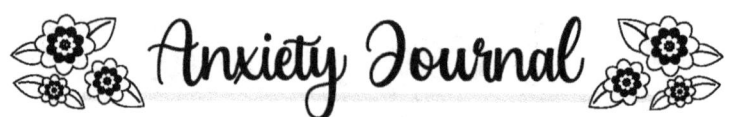
Anxiety Journal

DATE .... **TIME** ....

PLACE .... **SOURCE OF ANXIETY** ....

PHYSICAL SENSATIONS ....

NEGATIVE BELIEVES

ABOUT SITUATION ....
....

ABOUT YOUSELF ....
....

WHAT FACTS DO YOU KNOW ARE TRUE?

ABOUT SITUATION ....
....

ABOUT YOUSELF ....
....

WHAT HAPPENED?

....
....

HOW DID IT MAKE YOU FEEL?

....
....

HOW DID YOU REACT?

....
....

WHAT HELPS YOU SOOTHE YOUR ANXIETY?

....
....

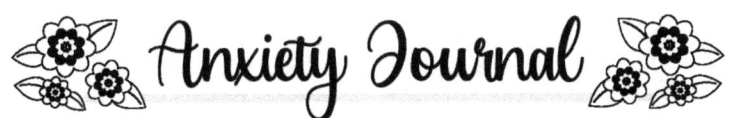

Anxiety Journal

DATE .... **TIME** ....

PLACE .... **SOURCE OF ANXIETY** ....

PHYSICAL SENSATIONS ....

NEGATIVE BELIEVES

ABOUT SITUATION ....
....

ABOUT YOUSELF ....
....

WHAT FACTS DO YOU KNOW ARE TRUE?

ABOUT SITUATION ....
....

ABOUT YOUSELF ....
....

WHAT HAPPENED?

....
....

HOW DID IT MAKE YOU FEEL?

....
....

HOW DID YOU REACT?

....
....

WHAT HELPS YOU SOOTHE YOUR ANXIETY?

....
....

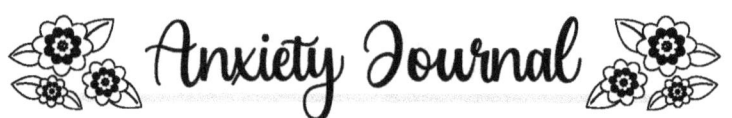
Anxiety Journal

DATE .... **TIME** ....

PLACE .... **SOURCE OF ANXIETY** ....

PHYSICAL SENSATIONS ....

NEGATIVE BELIEVES

ABOUT SITUATION ....
....

ABOUT YOUSELF ....
....

WHAT FACTS DO YOU KNOW ARE TRUE?

ABOUT SITUATION ....
....

ABOUT YOUSELF ....
....

WHAT HAPPENED?

....
....

HOW DID IT MAKE YOU FEEL?

....
....

HOW DID YOU REACT?

....
....

WHAT HELPS YOU SOOTHE YOUR ANXIETY?

....
....

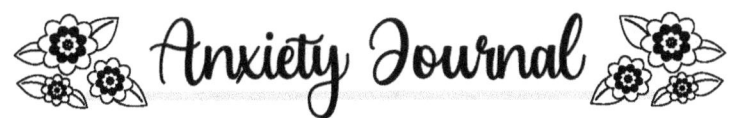 Anxiety Journal

DATE

TIME

PLACE

SOURCE OF ANXIETY

PHYSICAL SENSATIONS

NEGATIVE BELIEVES

ABOUT SITUATION ....

....

ABOUT YOUSELF ....

....

WHAT FACTS DO YOU KNOW ARE TRUE?

ABOUT SITUATION ....

....

ABOUT YOUSELF ....

....

WHAT HAPPENED?

....

....

HOW DID IT MAKE YOU FEEL?

....

....

HOW DID YOU REACT?

....

....

WHAT HELPS YOU SOOTHE YOUR ANXIETY?

....

....

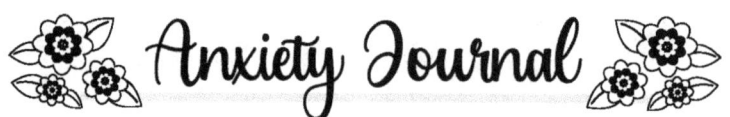

Anxiety Journal

DATE .... **TIME** ....

PLACE .... **SOURCE OF ANXIETY** ....

PHYSICAL SENSATIONS ....

NEGATIVE BELIEVES

ABOUT SITUATION ....
....

ABOUT YOUSELF ....
....

WHAT FACTS DO YOU KNOW ARE TRUE?

ABOUT SITUATION ....
....

ABOUT YOUSELF ....
....

WHAT HAPPENED?

....
....

HOW DID IT MAKE YOU FEEL?

....
....

HOW DID YOU REACT?

....
....

WHAT HELPS YOU SOOTHE YOUR ANXIETY?

....
....

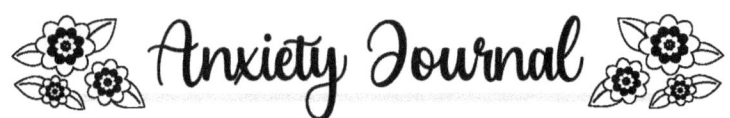

Anxiety Journal

DATE .... **TIME** ....

PLACE .... **SOURCE OF ANXIETY** ....

PHYSICAL SENSATIONS ....

NEGATIVE BELIEVES

ABOUT SITUATION ....
....

ABOUT YOUSELF ....
....

WHAT FACTS DO YOU KNOW ARE TRUE?

ABOUT SITUATION ....
....

ABOUT YOUSELF ....
....

WHAT HAPPENED?

....
....

HOW DID IT MAKE YOU FEEL?

....
....

HOW DID YOU REACT?

....
....

WHAT HELPS YOU SOOTHE YOUR ANXIETY?

....
....

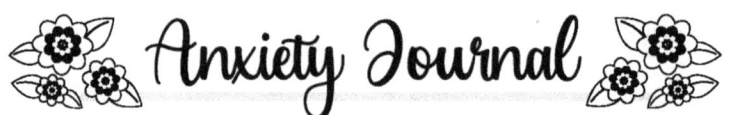

Anxiety Journal

DATE .... **TIME** ....

PLACE .... **SOURCE OF ANXIETY** ....

PHYSICAL SENSATIONS ....

NEGATIVE BELIEVES

ABOUT SITUATION ....
....

ABOUT YOUSELF ....
....

WHAT FACTS DO YOU KNOW ARE TRUE?

ABOUT SITUATION ....
....

ABOUT YOUSELF ....
....

WHAT HAPPENED?

....
....

HOW DID IT MAKE YOU FEEL?

....
....

HOW DID YOU REACT?

....
....

WHAT HELPS YOU SOOTHE YOUR ANXIETY?

....
....

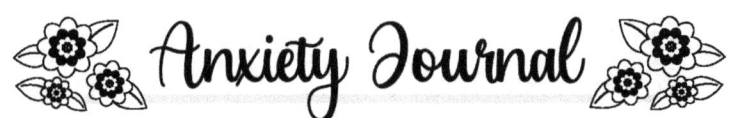
Anxiety Journal

DATE .... **TIME** ....

PLACE .... **SOURCE OF ANXIETY** ....

PHYSICAL SENSATIONS ....

NEGATIVE BELIEVES

ABOUT SITUATION ....
....

ABOUT YOUSELF ....
....

WHAT FACTS DO YOU KNOW ARE TRUE?

ABOUT SITUATION ....
....

ABOUT YOUSELF ....
....

WHAT HAPPENED?

....
....

HOW DID IT MAKE YOU FEEL?

....
....

HOW DID YOU REACT?

....
....

WHAT HELPS YOU SOOTHE YOUR ANXIETY?

....
....

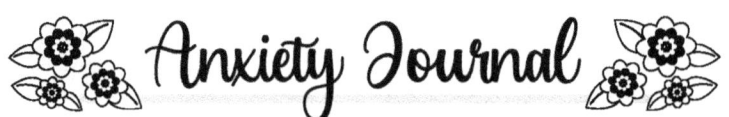

Anxiety Journal

DATE _____ **TIME** _____

PLACE _____ **SOURCE OF ANXIETY** _____

PHYSICAL SENSATIONS _____

NEGATIVE BELIEVES

ABOUT SITUATION ....
....

ABOUT YOUSELF ....
....

WHAT FACTS DO YOU KNOW ARE TRUE?

ABOUT SITUATION ....
....

ABOUT YOUSELF ....
....

WHAT HAPPENED?

....
....

HOW DID IT MAKE YOU FEEL?

....
....

HOW DID YOU REACT?

....
....

WHAT HELPS YOU SOOTHE YOUR ANXIETY?

....
....

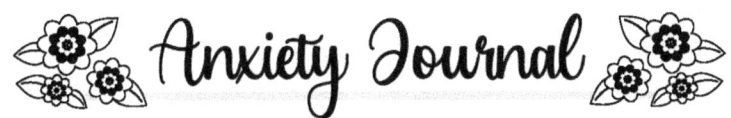

Anxiety Journal

DATE .... **TIME** ....

PLACE .... **SOURCE OF ANXIETY** ....

PHYSICAL SENSATIONS ....

NEGATIVE BELIEVES

ABOUT SITUATION ....

....

ABOUT YOUSELF ....

....

WHAT FACTS DO YOU KNOW ARE TRUE?

ABOUT SITUATION ....

....

ABOUT YOUSELF ....

....

WHAT HAPPENED?

....

....

HOW DID IT MAKE YOU FEEL?

....

....

HOW DID YOU REACT?

....

....

WHAT HELPS YOU SOOTHE YOUR ANXIETY?

....

....

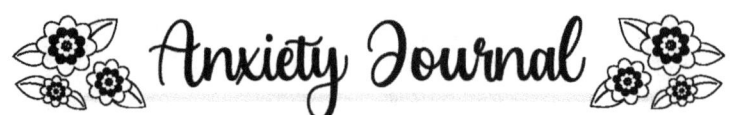

Anxiety Journal

DATE .... **TIME** ....

PLACE .... **SOURCE OF ANXIETY** ....

PHYSICAL SENSATIONS ....

NEGATIVE BELIEVES

ABOUT SITUATION ....
....

ABOUT YOUSELF ....
....

WHAT FACTS DO YOU KNOW ARE TRUE?

ABOUT SITUATION ....
....

ABOUT YOUSELF ....
....

WHAT HAPPENED?

....
....

HOW DID IT MAKE YOU FEEL?

....
....

HOW DID YOU REACT?

....
....

WHAT HELPS YOU SOOTHE YOUR ANXIETY?

....
....

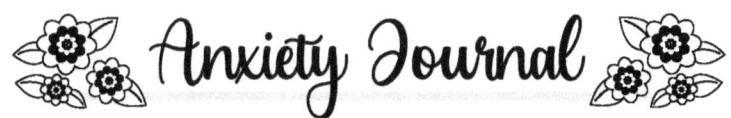

Anxiety Journal

DATE .... TIME ....

PLACE .... SOURCE OF ANXIETY ....

PHYSICAL SENSATIONS ....

NEGATIVE BELIEVES

ABOUT SITUATION ....
....

ABOUT YOUSELF ....
....

WHAT FACTS DO YOU KNOW ARE TRUE?

ABOUT SITUATION ....
....

ABOUT YOUSELF ....
....

WHAT HAPPENED?

....
....

HOW DID IT MAKE YOU FEEL?

....
....

HOW DID YOU REACT?

....
....

WHAT HELPS YOU SOOTHE YOUR ANXIETY?

....
....

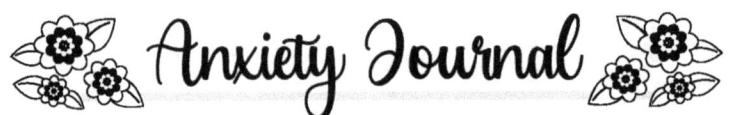

Anxiety Journal

DATE .... TIME ....

PLACE .... SOURCE OF ANXIETY ....

PHYSICAL SENSATIONS ....

NEGATIVE BELIEVES

ABOUT SITUATION ....

....

ABOUT YOUSELF ....

....

WHAT FACTS DO YOU KNOW ARE TRUE?

ABOUT SITUATION ....

....

ABOUT YOUSELF ....

....

WHAT HAPPENED?

....

....

HOW DID IT MAKE YOU FEEL?

....

....

HOW DID YOU REACT?

....

....

WHAT HELPS YOU SOOTHE YOUR ANXIETY?

....

....

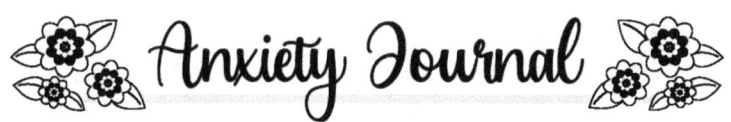

Anxiety Journal

DATE _____ **TIME** _____

PLACE _____ **SOURCE OF ANXIETY** _____

PHYSICAL SENSATIONS _____

NEGATIVE BELIEVES

ABOUT SITUATION ....
....

ABOUT YOUSELF ....
....

WHAT FACTS DO YOU KNOW ARE TRUE?

ABOUT SITUATION ....
....

ABOUT YOUSELF ....
....

WHAT HAPPENED?

....
....

HOW DID IT MAKE YOU FEEL?

....
....

HOW DID YOU REACT?

....
....

WHAT HELPS YOU SOOTHE YOUR ANXIETY?

....
....

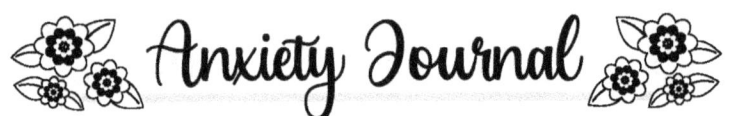

Anxiety Journal

DATE .... **TIME** ....

PLACE .... **SOURCE OF ANXIETY** ....

PHYSICAL SENSATIONS ....

NEGATIVE BELIEVES

ABOUT SITUATION ....

....

ABOUT YOUSELF ....

....

WHAT FACTS DO YOU KNOW ARE TRUE?

ABOUT SITUATION ....

....

ABOUT YOUSELF ....

....

WHAT HAPPENED?

....

....

HOW DID IT MAKE YOU FEEL?

....

....

HOW DID YOU REACT?

....

....

WHAT HELPS YOU SOOTHE YOUR ANXIETY?

....

....

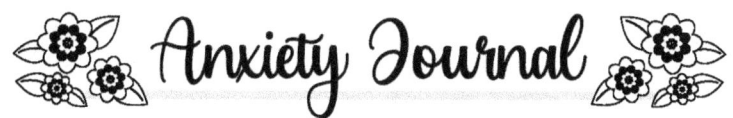

Anxiety Journal

DATE .... **TIME** ....

PLACE .... **SOURCE OF ANXIETY** ....

PHYSICAL SENSATIONS ....

NEGATIVE BELIEVES

ABOUT SITUATION ....
....

ABOUT YOUSELF ....
....

WHAT FACTS DO YOU KNOW ARE TRUE?

ABOUT SITUATION ....
....

ABOUT YOUSELF ....
....

WHAT HAPPENED?

....
....

HOW DID IT MAKE YOU FEEL?

....
....

HOW DID YOU REACT?

....
....

WHAT HELPS YOU SOOTHE YOUR ANXIETY?

....
....

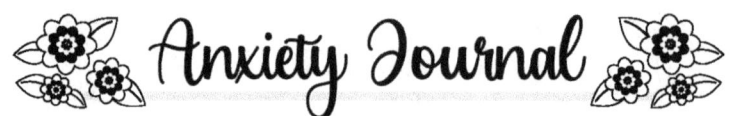

Anxiety Journal

DATE .... **TIME** ....

PLACE .... **SOURCE OF ANXIETY** ....

PHYSICAL SENSATIONS ....

NEGATIVE BELIEVES

ABOUT SITUATION ....
....

ABOUT YOUSELF ....
....

WHAT FACTS DO YOU KNOW ARE TRUE?

ABOUT SITUATION ....
....

ABOUT YOUSELF ....
....

WHAT HAPPENED?

....
....

HOW DID IT MAKE YOU FEEL?

....
....

HOW DID YOU REACT?

....
....

WHAT HELPS YOU SOOTHE YOUR ANXIETY?

....
....

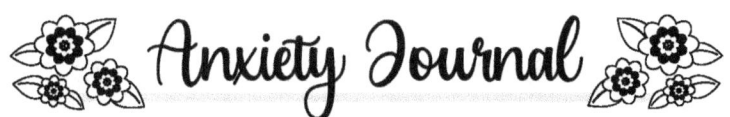

Anxiety Journal

DATE .... TIME ....

PLACE .... SOURCE OF ANXIETY ....

PHYSICAL SENSATIONS ....

NEGATIVE BELIEVES

ABOUT SITUATION ....
....

ABOUT YOUSELF ....
....

WHAT FACTS DO YOU KNOW ARE TRUE?

ABOUT SITUATION ....
....

ABOUT YOUSELF ....
....

WHAT HAPPENED?

....
....

HOW DID IT MAKE YOU FEEL?

....
....

HOW DID YOU REACT?

....
....

WHAT HELPS YOU SOOTHE YOUR ANXIETY?

....
....

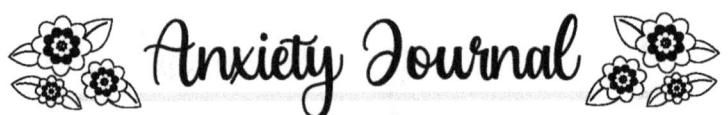

Anxiety Journal

DATE .... **TIME** ....

PLACE .... **SOURCE OF ANXIETY** ....

PHYSICAL SENSATIONS ....

NEGATIVE BELIEVES

ABOUT SITUATION ....

....

ABOUT YOUSELF ....

....

WHAT FACTS DO YOU KNOW ARE TRUE?

ABOUT SITUATION ....

....

ABOUT YOUSELF ....

....

WHAT HAPPENED?

....

....

HOW DID IT MAKE YOU FEEL?

....

....

HOW DID YOU REACT?

....

....

WHAT HELPS YOU SOOTHE YOUR ANXIETY?

....

....

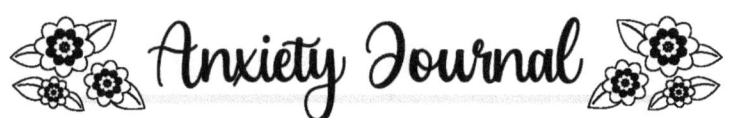

Anxiety Journal

DATE .... **TIME** ....

PLACE .... **SOURCE OF ANXIETY** ....

PHYSICAL SENSATIONS ....

NEGATIVE BELIEVES

ABOUT SITUATION ....
....

ABOUT YOUSELF ....
....

WHAT FACTS DO YOU KNOW ARE TRUE?

ABOUT SITUATION ....
....

ABOUT YOUSELF ....
....

WHAT HAPPENED?

....
....

HOW DID IT MAKE YOU FEEL?

....
....

HOW DID YOU REACT?

....
....

WHAT HELPS YOU SOOTHE YOUR ANXIETY?

....
....

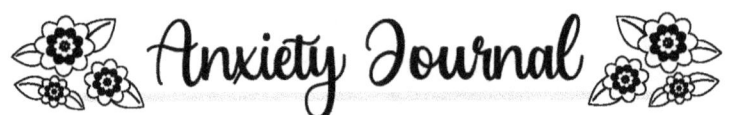

Anxiety Journal

DATE .... **TIME** ....

PLACE .... **SOURCE OF ANXIETY** ....

PHYSICAL SENSATIONS ....

NEGATIVE BELIEVES

ABOUT SITUATION ....
....

ABOUT YOUSELF ....
....

WHAT FACTS DO YOU KNOW ARE TRUE?

ABOUT SITUATION ....
....

ABOUT YOUSELF ....
....

WHAT HAPPENED?

....
....

HOW DID IT MAKE YOU FEEL?

....
....

HOW DID YOU REACT?

....
....

WHAT HELPS YOU SOOTHE YOUR ANXIETY?

....
....

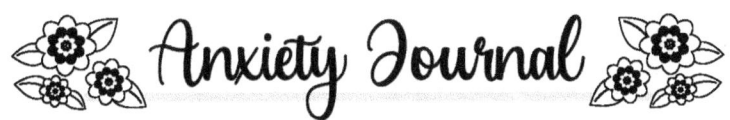

Anxiety Journal

DATE .... **TIME** ....

PLACE .... **SOURCE OF ANXIETY** ....

PHYSICAL SENSATIONS ....

NEGATIVE BELIEVES

ABOUT SITUATION ....
....

ABOUT YOUSELF ....
....

WHAT FACTS DO YOU KNOW ARE TRUE?

ABOUT SITUATION ....
....

ABOUT YOUSELF ....
....

WHAT HAPPENED?

....
....

HOW DID IT MAKE YOU FEEL?

....
....

HOW DID YOU REACT?

....
....

WHAT HELPS YOU SOOTHE YOUR ANXIETY?

....
....

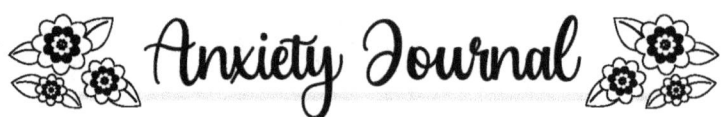

Anxiety Journal

DATE .... **TIME** ....

PLACE .... **SOURCE OF ANXIETY** ....

PHYSICAL SENSATIONS ....

NEGATIVE BELIEVES

ABOUT SITUATION ....
....

ABOUT YOUSELF ....
....

WHAT FACTS DO YOU KNOW ARE TRUE?

ABOUT SITUATION ....
....

ABOUT YOUSELF ....
....

WHAT HAPPENED?

....
....

HOW DID IT MAKE YOU FEEL?

....
....

HOW DID YOU REACT?

....
....

WHAT HELPS YOU SOOTHE YOUR ANXIETY?

....
....

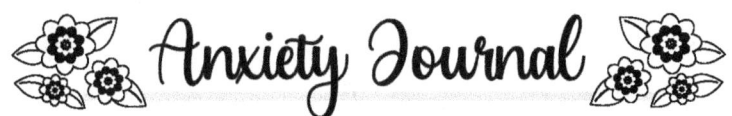

Anxiety Journal

DATE .... **TIME** ....

PLACE .... **SOURCE OF ANXIETY** ....

PHYSICAL SENSATIONS ....

NEGATIVE BELIEVES

ABOUT SITUATION ....
....

ABOUT YOUSELF ....
....

WHAT FACTS DO YOU KNOW ARE TRUE?

ABOUT SITUATION ....
....

ABOUT YOUSELF ....
....

WHAT HAPPENED?

....
....

HOW DID IT MAKE YOU FEEL?

....
....

HOW DID YOU REACT?

....
....

WHAT HELPS YOU SOOTHE YOUR ANXIETY?

....
....

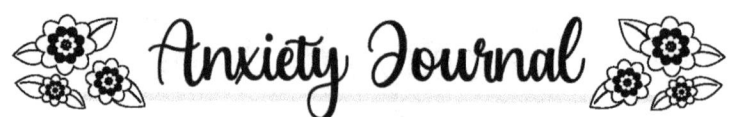

Anxiety Journal

DATE ....   TIME ....

PLACE ....   SOURCE OF ANXIETY ....

PHYSICAL SENSATIONS ....

NEGATIVE BELIEVES

ABOUT SITUATION ....
....

ABOUT YOUSELF ....
....

WHAT FACTS DO YOU KNOW ARE TRUE?

ABOUT SITUATION ....
....

ABOUT YOUSELF ....
....

WHAT HAPPENED?

....
....

HOW DID IT MAKE YOU FEEL?

....
....

HOW DID YOU REACT?

....
....

WHAT HELPS YOU SOOTHE YOUR ANXIETY?

....
....

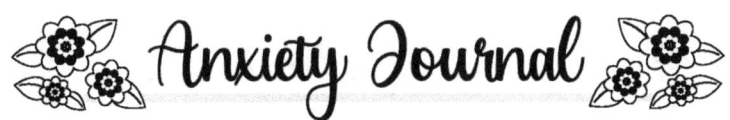

Anxiety Journal

DATE

TIME

PLACE

SOURCE OF ANXIETY

PHYSICAL SENSATIONS

NEGATIVE BELIEVES

ABOUT SITUATION ....

....

ABOUT YOUSELF ....

....

WHAT FACTS DO YOU KNOW ARE TRUE?

ABOUT SITUATION ....

....

ABOUT YOUSELF ....

....

WHAT HAPPENED?

....

....

HOW DID IT MAKE YOU FEEL?

....

....

HOW DID YOU REACT?

....

....

WHAT HELPS YOU SOOTHE YOUR ANXIETY?

....

....

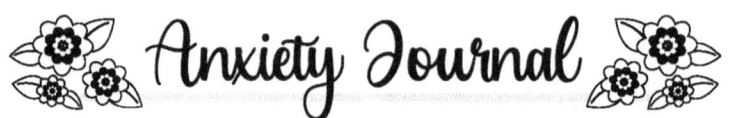

Anxiety Journal

DATE

TIME

PLACE

SOURCE OF ANXIETY

PHYSICAL SENSATIONS

NEGATIVE BELIEVES

ABOUT SITUATION ....

....

ABOUT YOUSELF ....

....

WHAT FACTS DO YOU KNOW ARE TRUE?

ABOUT SITUATION ....

....

ABOUT YOUSELF ....

....

WHAT HAPPENED?

....

....

HOW DID IT MAKE YOU FEEL?

....

....

HOW DID YOU REACT?

....

....

WHAT HELPS YOU SOOTHE YOUR ANXIETY?

....

....

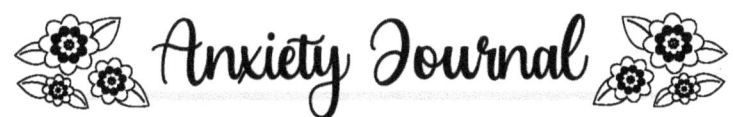

Anxiety Journal

DATE .... **TIME** ....

PLACE .... **SOURCE OF ANXIETY** ....

PHYSICAL SENSATIONS ....

NEGATIVE BELIEVES

ABOUT SITUATION ....

....

ABOUT YOUSELF ....

....

WHAT FACTS DO YOU KNOW ARE TRUE?

ABOUT SITUATION ....

....

ABOUT YOUSELF ....

....

WHAT HAPPENED?

....

....

HOW DID IT MAKE YOU FEEL?

....

....

HOW DID YOU REACT?

....

....

WHAT HELPS YOU SOOTHE YOUR ANXIETY?

....

....

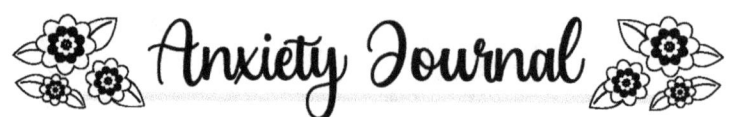

Anxiety Journal

DATE .... **TIME** ....

PLACE .... **SOURCE OF ANXIETY** ....

PHYSICAL SENSATIONS ....

NEGATIVE BELIEVES

ABOUT SITUATION ....
....

ABOUT YOUSELF ....
....

WHAT FACTS DO YOU KNOW ARE TRUE?

ABOUT SITUATION ....
....

ABOUT YOUSELF ....
....

WHAT HAPPENED?

....
....

HOW DID IT MAKE YOU FEEL?

....
....

HOW DID YOU REACT?

....
....

WHAT HELPS YOU SOOTHE YOUR ANXIETY?

....
....

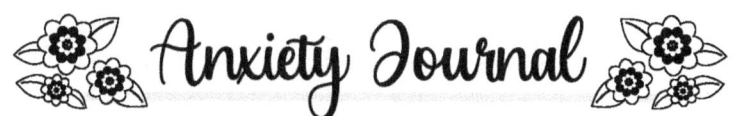

Anxiety Journal

DATE _____ **TIME** _____

PLACE _____ **SOURCE OF ANXIETY** _____

PHYSICAL SENSATIONS _____

NEGATIVE BELIEVES

ABOUT SITUATION ....
....

ABOUT YOUSELF ....
....

WHAT FACTS DO YOU KNOW ARE TRUE?

ABOUT SITUATION ....
....

ABOUT YOUSELF ....
....

WHAT HAPPENED?

....
....

HOW DID IT MAKE YOU FEEL?

....
....

HOW DID YOU REACT?

....
....

WHAT HELPS YOU SOOTHE YOUR ANXIETY?

....
....

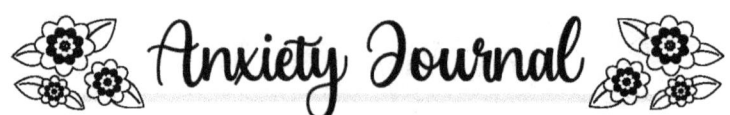

Anxiety Journal

DATE

TIME

PLACE

SOURCE OF ANXIETY

PHYSICAL SENSATIONS

NEGATIVE BELIEVES

ABOUT SITUATION ....
....

ABOUT YOUSELF ....
....

WHAT FACTS DO YOU KNOW ARE TRUE?

ABOUT SITUATION ....
....

ABOUT YOUSELF ....
....

WHAT HAPPENED?

....
....

HOW DID IT MAKE YOU FEEL?

....
....

HOW DID YOU REACT?

....
....

WHAT HELPS YOU SOOTHE YOUR ANXIETY?

....
....

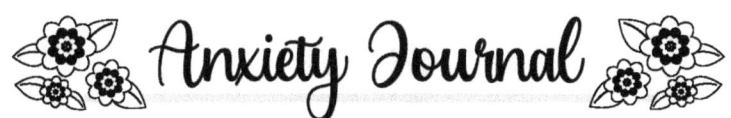

Anxiety Journal

DATE ....   **TIME** ....

PLACE ....   **SOURCE OF ANXIETY** ....

PHYSICAL SENSATIONS ....

NEGATIVE BELIEVES

ABOUT SITUATION ....

....

ABOUT YOUSELF ....

....

WHAT FACTS DO YOU KNOW ARE TRUE?

ABOUT SITUATION ....

....

ABOUT YOUSELF ....

....

WHAT HAPPENED?

....

....

HOW DID IT MAKE YOU FEEL?

....

....

HOW DID YOU REACT?

....

....

WHAT HELPS YOU SOOTHE YOUR ANXIETY?

....

....

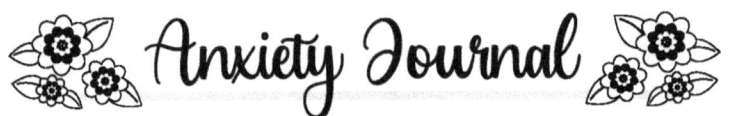

Anxiety Journal

DATE .... **TIME** ....

PLACE .... **SOURCE OF ANXIETY** ....

PHYSICAL SENSATIONS ....

NEGATIVE BELIEVES

ABOUT SITUATION ....

....

ABOUT YOUSELF ....

....

WHAT FACTS DO YOU KNOW ARE TRUE?

ABOUT SITUATION ....

....

ABOUT YOUSELF ....

....

WHAT HAPPENED?

....

....

HOW DID IT MAKE YOU FEEL?

....

....

HOW DID YOU REACT?

....

....

WHAT HELPS YOU SOOTHE YOUR ANXIETY?

....

....

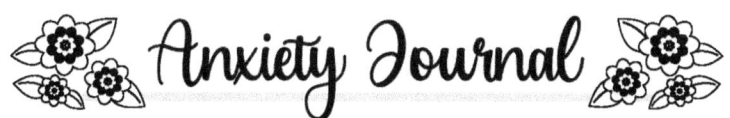
Anxiety Journal

DATE   **TIME**

PLACE   **SOURCE OF ANXIETY**

PHYSICAL SENSATIONS

NEGATIVE BELIEVES

ABOUT SITUATION ....
....

ABOUT YOUSELF ....
....

WHAT FACTS DO YOU KNOW ARE TRUE?

ABOUT SITUATION ....
....

ABOUT YOUSELF ....
....

WHAT HAPPENED?

....
....

HOW DID IT MAKE YOU FEEL?

....
....

HOW DID YOU REACT?

....
....

WHAT HELPS YOU SOOTHE YOUR ANXIETY?

....
....

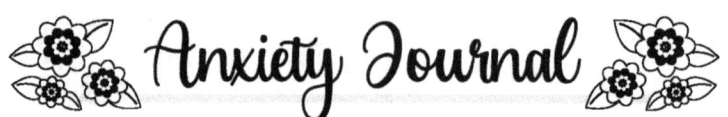
Anxiety Journal

DATE   **TIME**

PLACE   **SOURCE OF ANXIETY**

PHYSICAL SENSATIONS

NEGATIVE BELIEVES

ABOUT SITUATION ....
....

ABOUT YOUSELF ....
....

WHAT FACTS DO YOU KNOW ARE TRUE?

ABOUT SITUATION ....
....

ABOUT YOUSELF ....
....

WHAT HAPPENED?

....
....

HOW DID IT MAKE YOU FEEL?

....
....

HOW DID YOU REACT?

....
....

WHAT HELPS YOU SOOTHE YOUR ANXIETY?

....
....

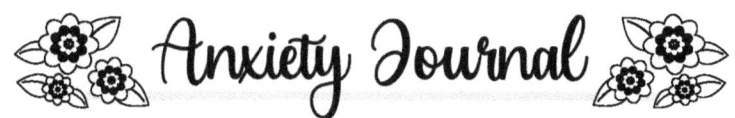

Anxiety Journal

DATE .... **TIME** ....

PLACE .... **SOURCE OF ANXIETY** ....

PHYSICAL SENSATIONS ....

NEGATIVE BELIEVES

ABOUT SITUATION ....
....

ABOUT YOUSELF ....
....

WHAT FACTS DO YOU KNOW ARE TRUE?

ABOUT SITUATION ....
....

ABOUT YOUSELF ....
....

WHAT HAPPENED?

....
....

HOW DID IT MAKE YOU FEEL?

....
....

HOW DID YOU REACT?

....
....

WHAT HELPS YOU SOOTHE YOUR ANXIETY?

....
....

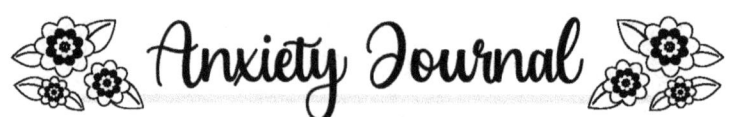

Anxiety Journal

DATE _____ **TIME** _____

PLACE _____ **SOURCE OF ANXIETY** _____

PHYSICAL SENSATIONS _____

NEGATIVE BELIEVES

ABOUT SITUATION ....

....

ABOUT YOUSELF ....

....

WHAT FACTS DO YOU KNOW ARE TRUE?

ABOUT SITUATION ....

....

ABOUT YOUSELF ....

....

WHAT HAPPENED?

....

....

HOW DID IT MAKE YOU FEEL?

....

....

HOW DID YOU REACT?

....

....

WHAT HELPS YOU SOOTHE YOUR ANXIETY?

....

....

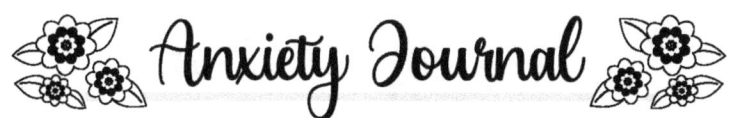

Anxiety Journal

DATE .... **TIME** ....

PLACE .... **SOURCE OF ANXIETY** ....

PHYSICAL SENSATIONS ....

NEGATIVE BELIEVES

ABOUT SITUATION ....

....

ABOUT YOUSELF ....

....

WHAT FACTS DO YOU KNOW ARE TRUE?

ABOUT SITUATION ....

....

ABOUT YOUSELF ....

....

WHAT HAPPENED?

....

....

HOW DID IT MAKE YOU FEEL?

....

....

HOW DID YOU REACT?

....

....

WHAT HELPS YOU SOOTHE YOUR ANXIETY?

....

....

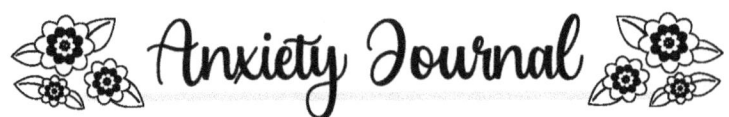
Anxiety Journal

DATE _____ **TIME** _____

PLACE _____ **SOURCE OF ANXIETY** _____

PHYSICAL SENSATIONS _____

NEGATIVE BELIEVES

ABOUT SITUATION ....
....

ABOUT YOUSELF ....
....

WHAT FACTS DO YOU KNOW ARE TRUE?

ABOUT SITUATION ....
....

ABOUT YOUSELF ....
....

WHAT HAPPENED?

....
....

HOW DID IT MAKE YOU FEEL?

....
....

HOW DID YOU REACT?

....
....

WHAT HELPS YOU SOOTHE YOUR ANXIETY?

....
....

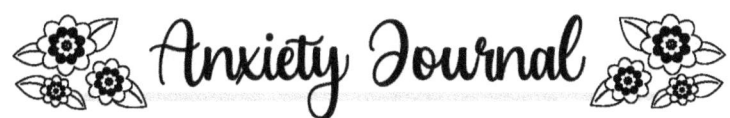

Anxiety Journal

DATE .... **TIME** ....

PLACE .... **SOURCE OF ANXIETY** ....

PHYSICAL SENSATIONS ....

NEGATIVE BELIEVES

ABOUT SITUATION ....
....

ABOUT YOUSELF ....
....

WHAT FACTS DO YOU KNOW ARE TRUE?

ABOUT SITUATION ....
....

ABOUT YOUSELF ....
....

WHAT HAPPENED?

....
....

HOW DID IT MAKE YOU FEEL?

....
....

HOW DID YOU REACT?

....
....

WHAT HELPS YOU SOOTHE YOUR ANXIETY?

....
....

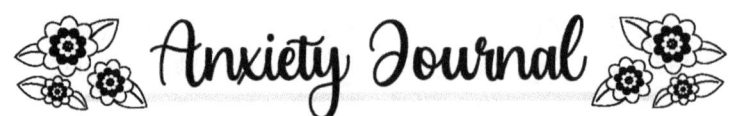

Anxiety Journal

DATE .... TIME ....

PLACE .... SOURCE OF ANXIETY ....

PHYSICAL SENSATIONS ....

NEGATIVE BELIEVES

ABOUT SITUATION ....
....

ABOUT YOUSELF ....
....

WHAT FACTS DO YOU KNOW ARE TRUE?

ABOUT SITUATION ....
....

ABOUT YOUSELF ....
....

WHAT HAPPENED?

....
....

HOW DID IT MAKE YOU FEEL?

....
....

HOW DID YOU REACT?

....
....

WHAT HELPS YOU SOOTHE YOUR ANXIETY?

....
....

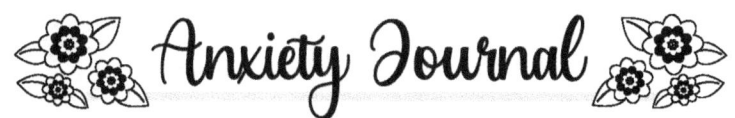

Anxiety Journal

DATE .... **TIME** ....

PLACE .... **SOURCE OF ANXIETY** ....

PHYSICAL SENSATIONS ....

NEGATIVE BELIEVES

ABOUT SITUATION ....
....

ABOUT YOUSELF ....
....

WHAT FACTS DO YOU KNOW ARE TRUE?

ABOUT SITUATION ....
....

ABOUT YOUSELF ....
....

WHAT HAPPENED?

....
....

HOW DID IT MAKE YOU FEEL?

....
....

HOW DID YOU REACT?

....
....

WHAT HELPS YOU SOOTHE YOUR ANXIETY?

....
....

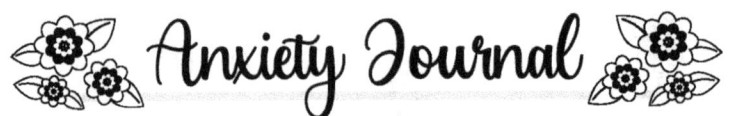

Anxiety Journal

DATE .... **TIME** ....

PLACE .... **SOURCE OF ANXIETY** ....

PHYSICAL SENSATIONS ....

NEGATIVE BELIEVES

ABOUT SITUATION ....
....

ABOUT YOUSELF ....
....

WHAT FACTS DO YOU KNOW ARE TRUE?

ABOUT SITUATION ....
....

ABOUT YOUSELF ....
....

WHAT HAPPENED?

....
....

HOW DID IT MAKE YOU FEEL?

....
....

HOW DID YOU REACT?

....
....

WHAT HELPS YOU SOOTHE YOUR ANXIETY?

....
....

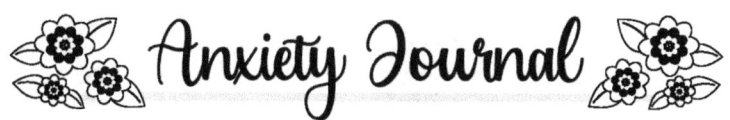
Anxiety Journal

DATE _____ **TIME** _____

PLACE _____ **SOURCE OF ANXIETY** _____

PHYSICAL SENSATIONS _____

NEGATIVE BELIEVES

ABOUT SITUATION ....

....

ABOUT YOUSELF ....

....

WHAT FACTS DO YOU KNOW ARE TRUE?

ABOUT SITUATION ....

....

ABOUT YOUSELF ....

....

WHAT HAPPENED?

....

....

HOW DID IT MAKE YOU FEEL?

....

....

HOW DID YOU REACT?

....

....

WHAT HELPS YOU SOOTHE YOUR ANXIETY?

....

....

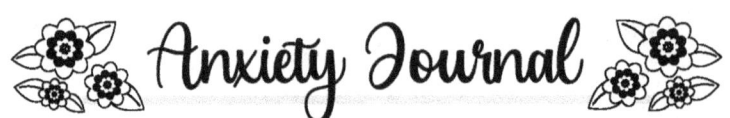

Anxiety Journal

DATE .... TIME ....

PLACE .... SOURCE OF ANXIETY ....

PHYSICAL SENSATIONS ....

NEGATIVE BELIEVES

ABOUT SITUATION ....

....

ABOUT YOUSELF ....

....

WHAT FACTS DO YOU KNOW ARE TRUE?

ABOUT SITUATION ....

....

ABOUT YOUSELF ....

....

WHAT HAPPENED?

....

....

HOW DID IT MAKE YOU FEEL?

....

....

HOW DID YOU REACT?

....

....

WHAT HELPS YOU SOOTHE YOUR ANXIETY?

....

....

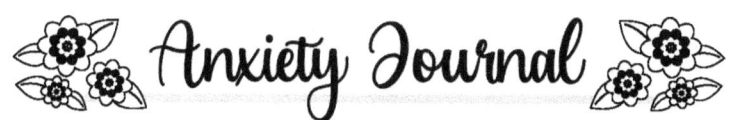

Anxiety Journal

DATE .... **TIME** ....

PLACE .... **SOURCE OF ANXIETY** ....

PHYSICAL SENSATIONS ....

NEGATIVE BELIEVES

ABOUT SITUATION ....

....

ABOUT YOUSELF ....

....

WHAT FACTS DO YOU KNOW ARE TRUE?

ABOUT SITUATION ....

....

ABOUT YOUSELF ....

....

WHAT HAPPENED?

....

....

HOW DID IT MAKE YOU FEEL?

....

....

HOW DID YOU REACT?

....

....

WHAT HELPS YOU SOOTHE YOUR ANXIETY?

....

....

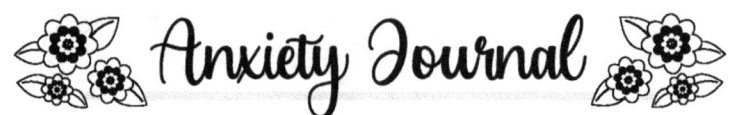

Anxiety Journal

DATE .... TIME ....

PLACE .... SOURCE OF ANXIETY ....

PHYSICAL SENSATIONS ....

NEGATIVE BELIEVES

ABOUT SITUATION ....

....

ABOUT YOUSELF ....

....

WHAT FACTS DO YOU KNOW ARE TRUE?

ABOUT SITUATION ....

....

ABOUT YOUSELF ....

....

WHAT HAPPENED?

....

....

HOW DID IT MAKE YOU FEEL?

....

....

HOW DID YOU REACT?

....

....

WHAT HELPS YOU SOOTHE YOUR ANXIETY?

....

....

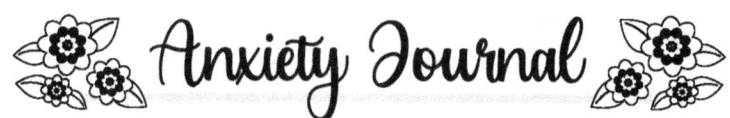

Anxiety Journal

DATE .... **TIME** ....

PLACE .... **SOURCE OF ANXIETY** ....

PHYSICAL SENSATIONS ....

NEGATIVE BELIEVES

ABOUT SITUATION ....
....

ABOUT YOUSELF ....
....

WHAT FACTS DO YOU KNOW ARE TRUE?

ABOUT SITUATION ....
....

ABOUT YOUSELF ....
....

WHAT HAPPENED?

....
....

HOW DID IT MAKE YOU FEEL?

....
....

HOW DID YOU REACT?

....
....

WHAT HELPS YOU SOOTHE YOUR ANXIETY?

....
....

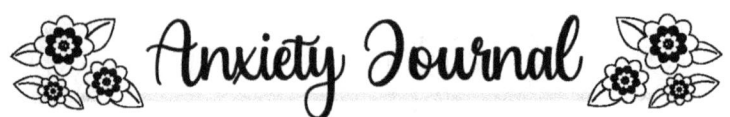
Anxiety Journal

DATE .... **TIME** ....

PLACE .... **SOURCE OF ANXIETY** ....

PHYSICAL SENSATIONS ....

NEGATIVE BELIEVES

ABOUT SITUATION ....
....

ABOUT YOUSELF ....
....

WHAT FACTS DO YOU KNOW ARE TRUE?

ABOUT SITUATION ....
....

ABOUT YOUSELF ....
....

WHAT HAPPENED?

....
....

HOW DID IT MAKE YOU FEEL?

....
....

HOW DID YOU REACT?

....
....

WHAT HELPS YOU SOOTHE YOUR ANXIETY?

....
....

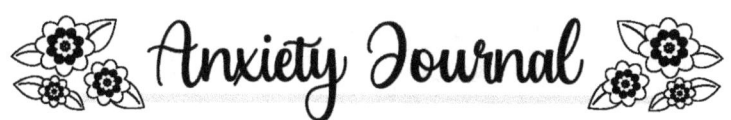

Anxiety Journal

DATE .... **TIME** ....

PLACE .... **SOURCE OF ANXIETY** ....

PHYSICAL SENSATIONS ....

NEGATIVE BELIEVES

ABOUT SITUATION ....

....

ABOUT YOUSELF ....

....

WHAT FACTS DO YOU KNOW ARE TRUE?

ABOUT SITUATION ....

....

ABOUT YOUSELF ....

....

WHAT HAPPENED?

....

....

HOW DID IT MAKE YOU FEEL?

....

....

HOW DID YOU REACT?

....

....

WHAT HELPS YOU SOOTHE YOUR ANXIETY?

....

....

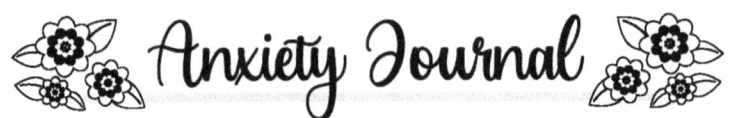
Anxiety Journal

DATE .... TIME ....

PLACE .... SOURCE OF ANXIETY ....

PHYSICAL SENSATIONS ....

NEGATIVE BELIEVES

ABOUT SITUATION ....

....

ABOUT YOUSELF ....

....

WHAT FACTS DO YOU KNOW ARE TRUE?

ABOUT SITUATION ....

....

ABOUT YOUSELF ....

....

WHAT HAPPENED?

....

....

HOW DID IT MAKE YOU FEEL?

....

....

HOW DID YOU REACT?

....

....

WHAT HELPS YOU SOOTHE YOUR ANXIETY?

....

....

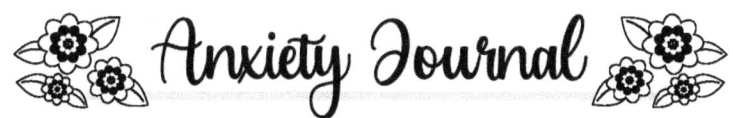

Anxiety Journal

DATE   **TIME**

PLACE   **SOURCE OF ANXIETY**

PHYSICAL SENSATIONS

NEGATIVE BELIEVES

ABOUT SITUATION ....
....

ABOUT YOUSELF ....
....

WHAT FACTS DO YOU KNOW ARE TRUE?

ABOUT SITUATION ....
....

ABOUT YOUSELF ....
....

WHAT HAPPENED?

....
....

HOW DID IT MAKE YOU FEEL?

....
....

HOW DID YOU REACT?

....
....

WHAT HELPS YOU SOOTHE YOUR ANXIETY?

....
....

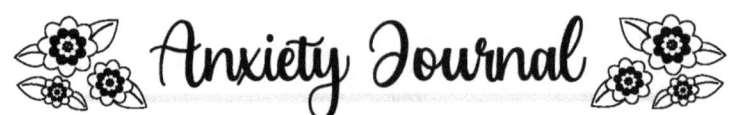

Anxiety Journal

DATE .... **TIME** ....

PLACE .... **SOURCE OF ANXIETY** ....

PHYSICAL SENSATIONS ....

NEGATIVE BELIEVES

ABOUT SITUATION ....
....

ABOUT YOUSELF ....
....

WHAT FACTS DO YOU KNOW ARE TRUE?

ABOUT SITUATION ....
....

ABOUT YOUSELF ....
....

WHAT HAPPENED?

....
....

HOW DID IT MAKE YOU FEEL?

....
....

HOW DID YOU REACT?

....
....

WHAT HELPS YOU SOOTHE YOUR ANXIETY?

....
....

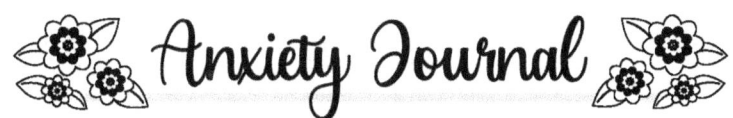

Anxiety Journal

DATE .... **TIME** ....

PLACE .... **SOURCE OF ANXIETY** ....

PHYSICAL SENSATIONS ....

NEGATIVE BELIEVES

ABOUT SITUATION ....
....

ABOUT YOUSELF ....
....

WHAT FACTS DO YOU KNOW ARE TRUE?

ABOUT SITUATION ....
....

ABOUT YOUSELF ....
....

WHAT HAPPENED?

....
....

HOW DID IT MAKE YOU FEEL?

....
....

HOW DID YOU REACT?

....
....

WHAT HELPS YOU SOOTHE YOUR ANXIETY?

....
....

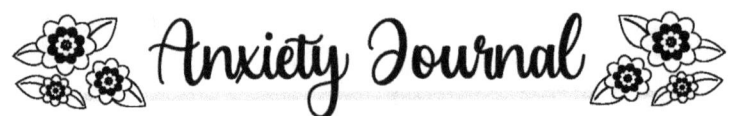

Anxiety Journal

DATE .... TIME ....

PLACE .... SOURCE OF ANXIETY ....

PHYSICAL SENSATIONS ....

NEGATIVE BELIEVES

ABOUT SITUATION ....

....

ABOUT YOUSELF ....

....

WHAT FACTS DO YOU KNOW ARE TRUE?

ABOUT SITUATION ....

....

ABOUT YOUSELF ....

....

WHAT HAPPENED?

....

....

HOW DID IT MAKE YOU FEEL?

....

....

HOW DID YOU REACT?

....

....

WHAT HELPS YOU SOOTHE YOUR ANXIETY?

....

....

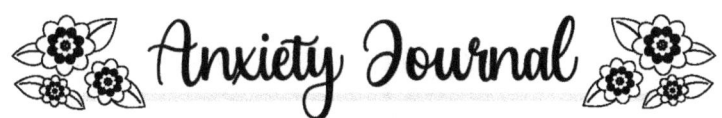

Anxiety Journal

DATE .... **TIME** ....

PLACE .... **SOURCE OF ANXIETY** ....

PHYSICAL SENSATIONS ....

NEGATIVE BELIEVES

ABOUT SITUATION ....
....

ABOUT YOUSELF ....
....

WHAT FACTS DO YOU KNOW ARE TRUE?

ABOUT SITUATION ....
....

ABOUT YOUSELF ....
....

WHAT HAPPENED?

....
....

HOW DID IT MAKE YOU FEEL?

....
....

HOW DID YOU REACT?

....
....

WHAT HELPS YOU SOOTHE YOUR ANXIETY?

....
....

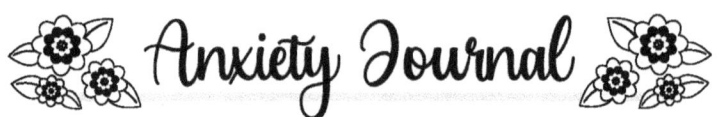

Anxiety Journal

DATE .... TIME ....

PLACE .... SOURCE OF ANXIETY ....

PHYSICAL SENSATIONS ....

NEGATIVE BELIEVES

ABOUT SITUATION ....
....

ABOUT YOUSELF ....
....

WHAT FACTS DO YOU KNOW ARE TRUE?

ABOUT SITUATION ....
....

ABOUT YOUSELF ....
....

WHAT HAPPENED?

....
....

HOW DID IT MAKE YOU FEEL?

....
....

HOW DID YOU REACT?

....
....

WHAT HELPS YOU SOOTHE YOUR ANXIETY?

....
....

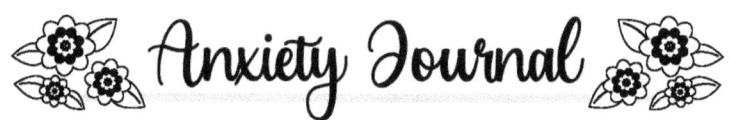

Anxiety Journal

DATE .... **TIME** ....

PLACE .... **SOURCE OF ANXIETY** ....

PHYSICAL SENSATIONS ....

NEGATIVE BELIEVES

ABOUT SITUATION ....

....

ABOUT YOUSELF ....

....

WHAT FACTS DO YOU KNOW ARE TRUE?

ABOUT SITUATION ....

....

ABOUT YOUSELF ....

....

WHAT HAPPENED?

....

....

HOW DID IT MAKE YOU FEEL?

....

....

HOW DID YOU REACT?

....

....

WHAT HELPS YOU SOOTHE YOUR ANXIETY?

....

....

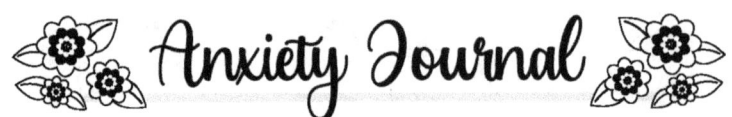

Anxiety Journal

DATE _____ **TIME** _____

PLACE _____ **SOURCE OF ANXIETY** _____

PHYSICAL SENSATIONS _____

NEGATIVE BELIEVES

ABOUT SITUATION ....
....

ABOUT YOUSELF ....
....

WHAT FACTS DO YOU KNOW ARE TRUE?

ABOUT SITUATION ....
....

ABOUT YOUSELF ....
....

WHAT HAPPENED?

....
....

HOW DID IT MAKE YOU FEEL?

....
....

HOW DID YOU REACT?

....
....

WHAT HELPS YOU SOOTHE YOUR ANXIETY?

....
....

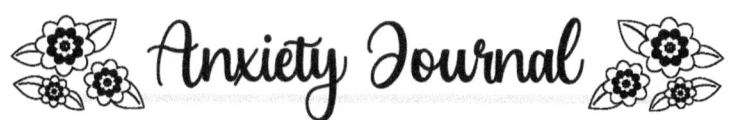

Anxiety Journal

DATE   **TIME**

PLACE   **SOURCE OF ANXIETY**

PHYSICAL SENSATIONS

NEGATIVE BELIEVES

ABOUT SITUATION ....

....

ABOUT YOUSELF ....

....

WHAT FACTS DO YOU KNOW ARE TRUE?

ABOUT SITUATION ....

....

ABOUT YOUSELF ....

....

WHAT HAPPENED?

....

....

HOW DID IT MAKE YOU FEEL?

....

....

HOW DID YOU REACT?

....

....

WHAT HELPS YOU SOOTHE YOUR ANXIETY?

....

....

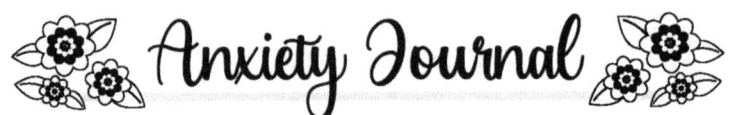

Anxiety Journal

DATE   **TIME**

PLACE   **SOURCE OF ANXIETY**

PHYSICAL SENSATIONS

NEGATIVE BELIEVES

ABOUT SITUATION ....
....

ABOUT YOUSELF ....
....

WHAT FACTS DO YOU KNOW ARE TRUE?

ABOUT SITUATION ....
....

ABOUT YOUSELF ....
....

WHAT HAPPENED?

....
....

HOW DID IT MAKE YOU FEEL?

....
....

HOW DID YOU REACT?

....
....

WHAT HELPS YOU SOOTHE YOUR ANXIETY?

....
....

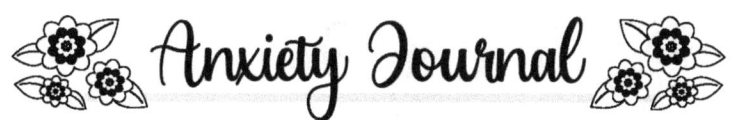# Anxiety Journal

DATE .... **TIME** ....

PLACE .... **SOURCE OF ANXIETY** ....

PHYSICAL SENSATIONS ....

NEGATIVE BELIEVES

ABOUT SITUATION ....
....

ABOUT YOUSELF ....
....

WHAT FACTS DO YOU KNOW ARE TRUE?

ABOUT SITUATION ....
....

ABOUT YOUSELF ....
....

WHAT HAPPENED?

....
....

HOW DID IT MAKE YOU FEEL?

....
....

HOW DID YOU REACT?

....
....

WHAT HELPS YOU SOOTHE YOUR ANXIETY?

....
....

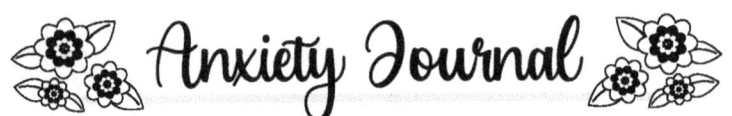
Anxiety Journal

DATE .... **TIME** ....

PLACE .... **SOURCE OF ANXIETY** ....

PHYSICAL SENSATIONS ....

NEGATIVE BELIEVES

ABOUT SITUATION ....
....

ABOUT YOUSELF ....
....

WHAT FACTS DO YOU KNOW ARE TRUE?

ABOUT SITUATION ....
....

ABOUT YOUSELF ....
....

WHAT HAPPENED?

....
....

HOW DID IT MAKE YOU FEEL?

....
....

HOW DID YOU REACT?

....
....

WHAT HELPS YOU SOOTHE YOUR ANXIETY?

....
....

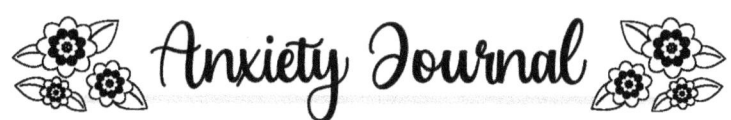

Anxiety Journal

DATE .... **TIME** ....

PLACE .... **SOURCE OF ANXIETY** ....

PHYSICAL SENSATIONS ....

NEGATIVE BELIEVES

ABOUT SITUATION ....
....

ABOUT YOUSELF ....
....

WHAT FACTS DO YOU KNOW ARE TRUE?

ABOUT SITUATION ....
....

ABOUT YOUSELF ....
....

WHAT HAPPENED?

....
....

HOW DID IT MAKE YOU FEEL?

....
....

HOW DID YOU REACT?

....
....

WHAT HELPS YOU SOOTHE YOUR ANXIETY?

....
....

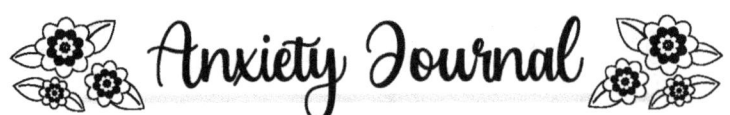 Anxiety Journal

DATE .... TIME ....

PLACE .... SOURCE OF ANXIETY ....

PHYSICAL SENSATIONS ....

NEGATIVE BELIEVES

ABOUT SITUATION ....

....

ABOUT YOUSELF ....

....

WHAT FACTS DO YOU KNOW ARE TRUE?

ABOUT SITUATION ....

....

ABOUT YOUSELF ....

....

WHAT HAPPENED?

....

....

HOW DID IT MAKE YOU FEEL?

....

....

HOW DID YOU REACT?

....

....

WHAT HELPS YOU SOOTHE YOUR ANXIETY?

....

....

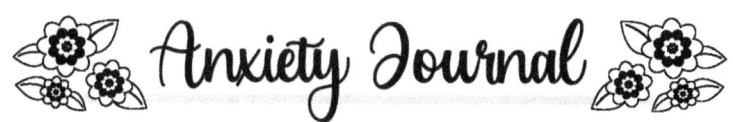

Anxiety Journal

DATE .... TIME ....

PLACE .... SOURCE OF ANXIETY ....

PHYSICAL SENSATIONS ....

NEGATIVE BELIEVES

ABOUT SITUATION ....
....

ABOUT YOUSELF ....
....

WHAT FACTS DO YOU KNOW ARE TRUE?

ABOUT SITUATION ....
....

ABOUT YOUSELF ....
....

WHAT HAPPENED?

....
....

HOW DID IT MAKE YOU FEEL?

....
....

HOW DID YOU REACT?

....
....

WHAT HELPS YOU SOOTHE YOUR ANXIETY?

....
....

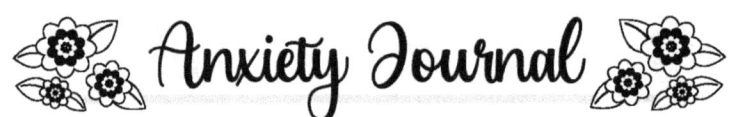 Anxiety Journal

DATE .... TIME ....

PLACE .... SOURCE OF ANXIETY ....

PHYSICAL SENSATIONS ....

NEGATIVE BELIEVES

ABOUT SITUATION ....
....

ABOUT YOUSELF ....
....

WHAT FACTS DO YOU KNOW ARE TRUE?

ABOUT SITUATION ....
....

ABOUT YOUSELF ....
....

WHAT HAPPENED?

....
....

HOW DID IT MAKE YOU FEEL?

....
....

HOW DID YOU REACT?

....
....

WHAT HELPS YOU SOOTHE YOUR ANXIETY?

....
....

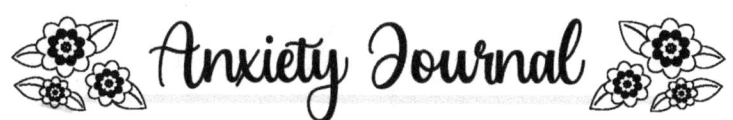

Anxiety Journal

DATE .... **TIME** ....

PLACE .... **SOURCE OF ANXIETY** ....

PHYSICAL SENSATIONS ....

NEGATIVE BELIEVES

ABOUT SITUATION ....
....

ABOUT YOUSELF ....
....

WHAT FACTS DO YOU KNOW ARE TRUE?

ABOUT SITUATION ....
....

ABOUT YOUSELF ....
....

WHAT HAPPENED?

....
....

HOW DID IT MAKE YOU FEEL?

....
....

HOW DID YOU REACT?

....
....

WHAT HELPS YOU SOOTHE YOUR ANXIETY?

....
....

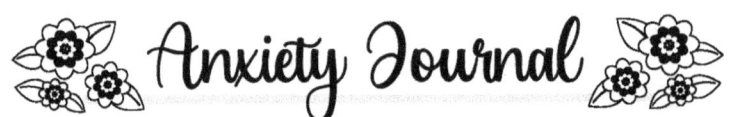
Anxiety Journal

DATE .... TIME ....

PLACE .... SOURCE OF ANXIETY ....

PHYSICAL SENSATIONS ....

NEGATIVE BELIEVES

ABOUT SITUATION ....
....

ABOUT YOUSELF ....
....

WHAT FACTS DO YOU KNOW ARE TRUE?

ABOUT SITUATION ....
....

ABOUT YOUSELF ....
....

WHAT HAPPENED?

....
....

HOW DID IT MAKE YOU FEEL?

....
....

HOW DID YOU REACT?

....
....

WHAT HELPS YOU SOOTHE YOUR ANXIETY?

....
....

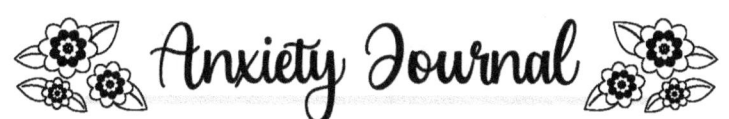

Anxiety Journal

DATE .... TIME ....

PLACE .... SOURCE OF ANXIETY ....

PHYSICAL SENSATIONS ....

NEGATIVE BELIEVES

ABOUT SITUATION ....
....

ABOUT YOUSELF ....
....

WHAT FACTS DO YOU KNOW ARE TRUE?

ABOUT SITUATION ....
....

ABOUT YOUSELF ....
....

WHAT HAPPENED?

....
....

HOW DID IT MAKE YOU FEEL?

....
....

HOW DID YOU REACT?

....
....

WHAT HELPS YOU SOOTHE YOUR ANXIETY?

....
....

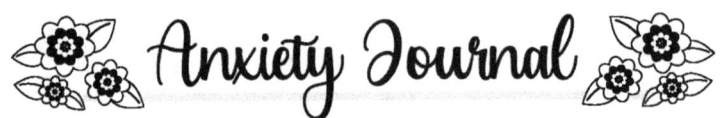

Anxiety Journal

DATE .... TIME ....

PLACE .... SOURCE OF ANXIETY ....

PHYSICAL SENSATIONS ....

NEGATIVE BELIEVES

ABOUT SITUATION ....
....

ABOUT YOUSELF ....
....

WHAT FACTS DO YOU KNOW ARE TRUE?

ABOUT SITUATION ....
....

ABOUT YOUSELF ....
....

WHAT HAPPENED?

....
....

HOW DID IT MAKE YOU FEEL?

....
....

HOW DID YOU REACT?

....
....

WHAT HELPS YOU SOOTHE YOUR ANXIETY?

....
....

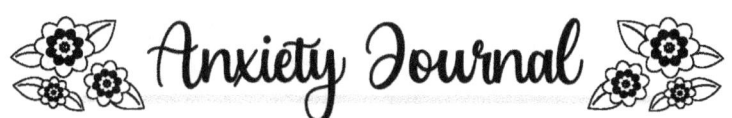

Anxiety Journal

DATE .... TIME ....

PLACE .... SOURCE OF ANXIETY ....

PHYSICAL SENSATIONS ....

NEGATIVE BELIEVES

ABOUT SITUATION ....

....

ABOUT YOUSELF ....

....

WHAT FACTS DO YOU KNOW ARE TRUE?

ABOUT SITUATION ....

....

ABOUT YOUSELF ....

....

WHAT HAPPENED?

....

....

HOW DID IT MAKE YOU FEEL?

....

....

HOW DID YOU REACT?

....

....

WHAT HELPS YOU SOOTHE YOUR ANXIETY?

....

....

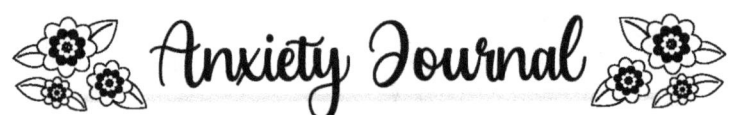

Anxiety Journal

DATE .... TIME ....

PLACE .... SOURCE OF ANXIETY ....

PHYSICAL SENSATIONS ....

NEGATIVE BELIEVES

ABOUT SITUATION ....
....

ABOUT YOUSELF ....
....

WHAT FACTS DO YOU KNOW ARE TRUE?

ABOUT SITUATION ....
....

ABOUT YOUSELF ....
....

WHAT HAPPENED?

....
....

HOW DID IT MAKE YOU FEEL?

....
....

HOW DID YOU REACT?

....
....

WHAT HELPS YOU SOOTHE YOUR ANXIETY?

....
....

CPSIA information can be obtained
at www.ICGtesting.com
Printed in the USA
BVHW041258160221
600147BV00031B/1860